Wrinkles:
Hair Growth:

Natural Home Remedies For Skin Care & Anti Aging; Natural Hair Growth For Hair Loss

WRINKLE CREAM GUIDE FOR BEGINNERS

Anti-Aging Wrinkle Cream Recipes to Naturally Rejuvenate & Hydrate your Skin

SOFIE KING

Table of Contents

Introduction

I want to thank you and congratulate you for purchasing the book, *"**WRINKLE CREAM GUIDE FOR BEGINNERS**: Anti-Aging Wrinkle Cream Recipes to Naturally Rejuvenate & Hydrate Your Skin"*.

This book contains proven steps and strategies on how to create natural skin care products to prevent and minimize your wrinkles. You will be able to save money on great skin care without compromising on the results.

Thanks again for purchasing this book, I hope you enjoy it! Please take some time to stop by and LIKE our Facebook page:

https://www.facebook.com/joypublishing

With gratitude,

SOFIE KING

Chapter 1

How Wrinkles Form?

In order to understand how to take care of your skin better, you must understand how wrinkles and other signs of aging form. Many people think that wrinkles form due to dry skin, but this is a mistake. While dry skin can exacerbate the formation of wrinkles and can make them more visible, dry skin does not necessarily cause them. What happens is dry skin does not have enough of the natural skin oil or sebum whose purpose is to protect the skin from the elements like sun, cold and wind. Thus, those with dry skin can easily form wrinkles even at a young age.

Further, if someone already has wrinkles and has dry skin too, the lack of sebum causes the wrinkles to become more prominent. Sebum or other moisturizers can plump up the skin causing wrinkles to look less deep or prominent. This is why those with mature skin are encouraged to use rich or very emollient moisturizers. It might seem as if the moisturizer 'cures' the wrinkles, but they will soon be visible again once the moisture wears off or once that person washes her face.

Also, many think that only old people can get wrinkles. While this is true for most cases, some old folks can have youthful looking skin. Also, young people can get wrinkles if they do not properly take care of their skin. The signs of aging start to show by the age of 30, but this does not mean they have not started to accumulate as early as one's teenage years. If you spent most of your younger years under the sun without sun protection products or if you don't take care of your skin with proper nutrition or skin care products, the damage will accumulate deep in the skin's dermis layer and will show up by the time you reach your late 20s or early 30s. Those who spend their whole days under the sun since childhood might see signs of aging as early as their mid-20s.

What we must understand here is that skin damage slowly accumulates. If you spend only one day a year under the sun without sun protection products, your accumulated damage will be less compared to someone who spends every day under the sun.

Of course, unless you never go outside and never sit beside a clear window, and unless you live in a pristine environment with no hint of air or water pollution, you cannot escape from skin damage. Monks who live in dark monasteries can reach the age of 80 but still have the smooth and clear skin of a teenager. If living in the dark is not appealing to you, then rest assured that there are ways to prevent and minimize skin damage.

The skin accumulates damage due to UVA rays and free radicals in the environment. UVA rays or ultraviolet rays A are responsible for the majority of the signs of skin aging but most especially for the breakdown of collagen and elastin in the skin's dermis layer. These are the proteins necessary to keep the skin looking smooth, firm and bouncy.

While the body can replace damaged collagen, the natural aging process slows down the rejuvenating powers of the body. This is why a 20 year old who has experienced intense sun for a long period of time, e.g. a week's holiday at the beach, will have less damage than a 40 year old who has experienced the same.

It is also possible that the damage received on a daily basis is too much for the body to handle. A 20 year old who receives daily sun damage will probably have the same skin as a 40 year old who only receives sun damage in the form of his yearly beach trip.

UVAs can permeate even through clouds and thick but clear glass windows. Thick, tightly woven clothing can provide some protection but thin weaves will allow most of it to pass through. The other kind of ultraviolet ray, UVB, is responsible for tanning the skin. It does not cause as much damage to collagen and elastin but it can dry the skin and can contribute to an increased risk of developing skin cancer.

Moving on to free radicals, these are atoms or molecules with an unpaired electron in its outer shell. If you still remember your high school chemistry, you'll know that having an extra electron makes this atom or molecule unstable. It needs to join up with another atom or molecule from which it will 'steal' a proton. If it 'steals' protons from your skin cells, this will cause damage. While damage to one skin cell will not be significant, a lot of damage, especially if it accumulates over time, will result in an increase in wrinkles.

Free radicals are plentiful in polluted environments like cities or areas near factories. This is why people who live in these areas can look older than those who live in the country or in cleaner environments assuming they give their skin the same level of care. Free radicals can also enter the body through certain foods like junk food and excess sweets, but their effect will mostly be seen in other parts of the body like an impaired immune system and cancer of the internal organs. As far as the skin is concerned, most of the damage will come from air and water pollution when it comes into contact with the skin.

While free radicals can cause damage, it plays a small part in the formation of wrinkles. The sun still causes about 90% of the signs of aging with 10% caused by other factors. Thus, if someone lives in the country where the environment is clean but he is always out in the sun, he will have a lot of skin damage.

In addition to the sun and free radicals, we must include the destructive abilities of unhealthy habits like smoking, lack of proper nutrition and lack of sleep.

Smoking pours several poisons into the body which the body must try to remove if it does not want to die. The effort of cleansing the body of the poisons from cigarettes can tire it so much that it cannot focus on taking care of its various parts. This is why the immune system can weaken, the internal organs can become diseased and the skin becomes dull and sickly looking. If you are a young person whose body's rejuvenating powers are still at its peak, then your body can easily heal even if you smoke 2 packs a day, but only up to a certain point. By your mid-20s, the body might be too exhausted and slowly degenerate.

Regarding the lack of proper nutrition, the human body is an animal body and needs nourishment outside of itself. We need the various nutrients in their proper amounts to keep the body running. Even young people whose bodily functions are at their peak will soon break down if proper nutritional needs are not met.

Since the skin is part of the body, lack of nutrition will affect it. For example, vitamin A is necessary for the maintenance and repair of the skin. If your diet lacks it, your body might still have the ability to repair skin if you are still relatively young, but without the proper tools it will not do a very good job. To give an analogy, think of a skilled craftsman without the proper tools. He might be able to do the job but it will not be as good as when he has all the required tools.

Lastly, sleep is very important since this is the time when the body does its major repairs. Even if you are still young and eat properly, the lack of sleep does not give the body a chance to heal. Again, to give an analogy, this is like a skilled craftsman with the proper tools who is not given a break from work. Soon, tiredness will affect him and he will make mistakes that will affect the quality of his work.

Notice that there are several factors that cause skin damage and exacerbate it. You have to take all these things into consideration when determining how to prevent wrinkles. To summarize, here are the things that cause and exacerbate the signs of aging:

- UVA rays

- Free radicals

- Dry skin or the lack of sebum which acts as *some* protection against the sun, wind and cold.

- The body's lessened ability to regenerate itself which naturally happens due to aging. Generally speaking, the slowing down of the skin's ability to regenerate itself starts around the age of 30.

- Unhealthy habits like smoking, improper diet and lack of sleep.

These factors all contribute to the damaged collagen and elastin in the dermal layer of the skin. If the dermis is damaged, the epidermis follows the form of the damage. This shows up in the form of wrinkles.

Chapter 2

The Truth about Preventing Wrinkles

Now that we know what causes wrinkles, we can easily prevent it. Obviously, what we need to do is to avoid or minimize exposure to the causes listed above.

Since the sun causes 90% of skin damage, that is our number 1 concern. A variety of sun protection products exist in the market today to shield our skin from the UV rays, but most people don't know how to choose the best products. They also don't know how to properly use them.

In the first place, they choose a product according to the SPF (sun protection factor) number. That only indicates the amount of protection given against UVB rays. I am not saying that protecting yourself against UVB rays is bad, but as far as skin aging is concerned, you must focus on protecting yourself against UVA.

This is why it is more important to focus on the PA (protection against UVA) rating. You can know this according to the number of +'s indicated. PA+ gives you minimal protection and is best for those who only get about 10 minutes of sun. Those who are more exposed should look for PA++ or even PA+++.

In the second place, while people *do* apply sun protection, they do not apply enough. You need about 2 teaspoons of product for your whole face and neck and about 2 shot glassfuls for the whole body if you are going to expose most of your skin. If you are only going to expose your arms or hands, use a similar amount as you would for hand lotion.

You need to use these amounts to get the level of protection indicated in the package. If you don't then your SPF 15 might only be an SPF of 10 or 5. Also, don't skimp on sun protection even if you use make-up or moisturizers with SPF and PA. Since you don't use 2 teaspoons of these products on your face and neck, you are not using enough to provide adequate protection. The protection provided by these products is a good plus, but you must not solely depend on them.

Properly using sun protection products also means reapplying often. Ideally, you should reapply every 2 hours if you are under the sun, but if you have been sweating profusely or have been swimming, you should reapply immediately even if it has only been an hour. If you dislike reapplying throughout the day, you are better off using the highest level of protection you can find. Instead of 2 hours, you can get away with reapplying every 4 hours.

Now let us discuss the prevention of free radical damage. This can be avoided by applying topical skin care with antioxidants. The antioxidants protect the skin by attaching to the free radicals thus preventing them from attaching and damaging the skin cells.

The jury is still out regarding which antioxidant is best for the skin so don't worry too much about what to get. Instead, choose products according to your skin type and personal preference like fragrance, texture, packaging and the like.

You can also prevent free radical damage by eating your antioxidants. Increasing your intake of fresh fruits and vegetables, and other foods that are rich in antioxidants like tea, dark chocolate and red wine can all contribute to better skin. However, the difference between ingested and topical antioxidants is the latter can better protect the skin while the former will be directed to various parts of the body. After all, the body has several other organs it must take care of, but this is not to say that an increased intake of these good foods will not have an effect on the skin. As we have said, proper nutrition allows the body to function properly, including the repair of its damaged parts.

Regarding dry skin, as we have discussed previously, well-hydrated skin can better protect itself from the natural elements. We will discuss ways to hydrate the skin in the next chapter.

Regarding the body's lessened ability to regenerate itself, nothing can be done to prevent this, but something can be done to help the skin regenerate itself to minimize the effects of accumulated damage. We will discuss this further in chapter 4.

Lastly, when it comes to your unhealthy habits, it is your responsibility to take care of your body. If you smoke, stop. If you don't eat well, make an effort. If you don't sleep enough, rearrange your schedule to avoid too much work or make your bedroom more relaxing. If you are serious about taking care of your skin, you must become serious about taking care of your body. All the tips listed in this book will be for nothing if you still insist on your unhealthy habits.

Chapter 3

Recipes for Wrinkle Prevention

Here are some recipes for natural skin care products. They are a good substitute for commercially available products because they are cheaper in the long run. Also, you can tailor them according to your needs.

Before we discuss these recipes, we must mention some reminders when making products at home:

- Use a separate saucepan, mixers, bowls, etc. for your skin care products. You might need to use ingredients that are poisonous when ingested.

- Measure your ingredients well. Too much of an ingredient can cause irritation or will not result in a good product.

- Some ingredients are poisonous when inhaled. For safety reasons, use a mask when making these products.

- Use sterilized opaque glass containers for your finished products. You can sterilize them by pouring boiling water over them then leaving them to dry. Opaque glasses will help prevent their disintegration due to sunlight, but if you cannot find opaque glass containers, just keep your products in a dark place.

- If you live in a hot climate, it is best to store your natural products in the refrigerator, but make sure that no will suspect it for food. Label all products well and keep them out of children's reach.

- Buy ingredients from reputable sources. For example, make sure that you are buying fresh Shea or cocoa butter. Beeswax should be purified and free from bee bodies or traces of honey. Essential oils should be true oils and not artificial fragrance oils.

- If you have sensitive skin, always do a skin test before using any of these products. If you have extremely sensitive skin, it is best to stick to the commercially available products that have been tested for safety. Otherwise, those who are not so sensitive will generally not experience any irritation with the recipes listed in this book.

Sun Protection Cream

(This will give you SPF 20 and PA+, but you can add more zinc oxide to increase the level of protection. Doing this might make your cream leave a whitish cast that is especially obvious on dark skin. Experiment with the amount of zinc oxide that works best for you, but do not use less than 2 tablespoons for ½ cup of cream base.)

Ingredients:

- ¼ cup coconut, almond or jojoba oil (normal skin), or olive, argan or avocado oil (dry skin) or grape seed oil (oily skin)
- ¼ cup beeswax (normal or oily skin) or Shea or cocoa butter (dry skin)
- 2 tablespoons non-nano zinc oxide powder (do not inhale)

Procedure:

1. Melt the beeswax or Shea or cocoa butter in a saucepan.

2. Remove from the heat. Add the oil and mix well.

3. Add the zinc oxide and mix thoroughly.

4. Pour into your prepared container and allow to cool before using.

Antioxidant Toner

Ingredients:

- ½ cup strongly brewed green tea (use 1 tea bag in ½ cup of boiling water)
- 5 drops of green tea essential oil
  Optional: 2 drops of lemon, jasmine or lavender essential oil for fragrance

Procedure:

1. Once the tea is cooled, mix everything together in a glass bottle.

2. Use a cotton ball to apply. Shake well before every use.

Antioxidant Moisturizer

Ingredients:

- ¼ cup coconut, almond or jojoba oil (normal skin), or olive, argan or avocado oil (dry skin) or grape seed oil (oily skin)
- ¼ cup beeswax (normal or oily skin) or Shea or cocoa butter (dry skin)
- 10 drops of green tea essential oil
  Optional: 2 drops of lemon, jasmine or lavender essential oil for fragrance

Procedure:

Melt the beeswax or Shea or cocoa butter in a saucepan.

Remove from the heat. Add the oil and mix well.

Once it is well-mixed, add the essential oils and mix again.

Pour into your container and allow to cool before using.

Apply a pea sized amount all over the face and neck. If you used lavender essential oil, avoid applying near the eyes.

Basic Dry Skin Cream

(This can also be used for rough patches like elbows and knees.)

Ingredients:

- ¼ cup olive, argan or avocado oil
- ¼ cup Shea or cocoa butter

Procedure:

1. Melt the butter in a saucepan.

2. Remove from the heat and add the oil. Mix well.

3. Pour into your container and leave to cool.

Basic Dry Skin Facial Oil

(Facial oil is good for those who travel frequently. Since the oil is more emollient, you don't need much. A small amount will last you a long time. For extremely dry skin or during cold weather, apply the oil first then the cream. This oil can also be applied to dry hair and rough spots like elbows and knees.)

Ingredients:

- ¼ cup olive, argan, or avocado oil
- *Optional:* 2 drops of your choice of essential oil to add fragrance. Do not use lavender, peppermint or other similar scents if you wish to use this around your eye area.

Procedure:

1. Keep your oil in a bottle.

2. Add the essential oil and shake together to mix.

3. Use 1-2 drops of oil for moisturizing the whole face.

Rose Dry Skin Cream

(This has the natural feminine fragrance of roses. Do not use this if you are allergic to fragrance. Using fragranced products makes you look forward to using moisturizer. This is also a good choice for mature skin with deep wrinkles.)

Ingredients:

- 1 batch of basic dry skin cream
- 4 tablespoons of rosehip oil
- 5 drops of rose essential oil
  Optional: 2 drops of sandalwood essential oil (This will give your cream a more mature, sophisticated scent.)

Procedure:

1. Follow the steps in making the basic dry skin cream. Add the rosehip oil with the other oils.

2. After the rosehip oil is well-mixed, add the rose essential oil. Mix further then pour into your container.

Rose Dry Skin Facial Oil

Ingredients:

- 1 batch of basic dry skin facial oil
- 4 tablespoons rosehip oil
- 5 drops rose essential oil
  Optional: 2 drops of sandalwood essential oil

Procedure:

1. After making a batch of basic dry skin facial oil, add the other ingredients.

2. Shake well to mix.

Chapter 4

The Truth about 'Curing' Wrinkles

Now let us discuss what you have to do when you already have wrinkles. I have used the word 'cure' here but I only do this to prove a point about wrinkles. Once you have them, you cannot completely 'cure' them. What you can do is only to minimize their appearance, i.e. make them less deep. Thus, the truth about 'curing' wrinkles is this: it is impossible. The best way to keep your skin's youthful appearance is to prevent the signs of aging from showing up.

At this point you might say, 'But wait? What about those people with wrinkles who go through certain procedures and emerge looking youthful and fresh?'

Look at the before and after pictures closely. If the 'after' picture shows a person with an extremely youthful appearance, the 'before' picture likely shows a person without that much signs of skin aging, perhaps only a few shallow wrinkles around the eyes and mouth. The point here is you have to consider the starting point to understand how much improvement can be expected, and the answer will always be 'not 100%'.

Now you might think, 'but what about those who get a face lift?' The face lift stretches the skin so the wrinkles seem to smoothen, but that results in an unattractive 'tight faced' look. You have not actually cured the wrinkles but merely disguised them.

If this is the truth about 'curing' wrinkles, then what exactly can be done? 2 things can be done to 'cure' or minimize wrinkles: temporarily plumping the skin with moisturizer to disguise wrinkles, and forcing the skin to produce more collagen and elastin to make the wrinkles shallower. Now remember that since you cannot completely remove a wrinkle once it has formed, the collagen and elastin which certain skin care products can create will never be enough to bring your damaged skin back to its youthful glory, but at least the damage will be minimized.

First, let us discuss how to temporarily plump the skin. In chapter 1, we talked about how dry skin makes wrinkles more obvious because the skin is not plumped up. To give a rather obvious analogy, dry skin is like a raisin and adding moisturizer is like soaking that raisin in water. As the water gets into the raisin, it plumps up and its wrinkles become shallower.

To temporarily plump up the skin, you can use the dry skin cream or facial oil recipes described above or one of the commercially available products specifically made for dry skin. These products are extremely emollient and are designed to minimize water loss from the skin's cells. To increase the skin's water content, thus allowing it to look plumper, apply moisturizer on damp skin. In the middle of the day or whenever your skin feels dry, you can spritz some water on your face then apply more moisturizer.

You can do this even if you are wearing make-up, but you'll have to reapply more make-up since the moisturizer will dilute the colors. Just make sure that you only do this on a clean face, i.e. if you have been walking around a smoggy environment, you probably need to wash your face first instead of adding more moisturizer and make-up on top of that layer of dirt.

Second, let's consider how to permanently add more collagen and elastin to your skin. The only products that have been actually proven to significantly increase collagen and elastin are tretinoin and peptides. Tretinoin is more effective but can be very irritating if used daily. Peptides are less effective but are gentler to the skin. Those with sensitive skin can use a lower percentage of tretinoin and alternate it with peptides. Those with normal skin can probably use tretinoin every day.

While some products may advertise their ingredients as being clinically proven to do the same, this may only mean that they were shown to improve collagen and elastin in sample human skin cells in a laboratory but not necessarily in actual human skin.

You can buy skin care products with tretinoin or peptides from commercially available brands. Do not attempt to make your own. Besides, you will not be able to buy pure tretinoin or peptides as ingredients.

That said, there are still ways to increase collagen and elastin through natural beauty products like certain essential oils and plant oils. For example, rosehip oil is high in vitamin A and can give you similar effects as tretinoin which is also a form of vitamin A. Essential oils like lavender, sandalwood and patchouli can stimulate the capillaries in facial skin; thus bringing more blood to those areas that in turn means more nutrients.

However, their effects will not be as significant as tretinoin and peptides. You will probably need to wait a year of daily applications of rosehip oil to see the same results tretinoin can give in 4 months or peptides in 6. With regard to essential oils, they can only indirectly increase collagen and elastin by encouraging the body to bring more nutrients to the skin and thus give the cells what they need to repair themselves.

If you do not support this practice with proper nutrition and with adequate sleep, the increased blood brought to your facial skin will do nothing since it will not bring with it the skin's nutrients. You will also cancel out any good effects if you insist on the habit of smoking.

Another way to increase collagen and elastin is by regularly exfoliating the skin. By removing the top layer of the epidermis, you force the skin to reproduce more skin cells and repair itself. However, exfoliation will not make the skin produce the same amount of collagen and elastin as tretinoin and peptides will encourage it to.

Finally, the application of topical vitamin C can help to increase collagen and elastin production but only to a certain degree and not as much as the result of using tretinoin or peptides. Vitamin C is necessary in the production of these skin proteins so providing the skin with this nutrient encourages it to repair itself.

Chapter 5

Recipes for Deep Wrinkles

Though you cannot create tretinoin or peptide products on your own, you can still create products that stimulate collagen and elastin production even if only slightly. You can alternate between using tretinoin and/or peptides and essential oil moisturizers. Also, exfoliate your skin at least once a week for dry skin and twice a week for normal skin. Exfoliating will also minimize dark spots and reduce the dullness that is common in aging skin.

Essential Oil Wrinkle Reducing Cream

(This can be used at night while the antioxidant moisturizer can be used in the mornings before applying your sun protection product.)

Ingredients:

- ¼ cup coconut, almond or jojoba oil (normal skin), or olive, argan or avocado oil (dry skin) or grape seed oil (oily skin)
- ¼ cup beeswax (normal or oily skin) or shea or cocoa butter (dry skin)
- 10 drops of lavender, patchouli, sandalwood, chamomile or rose essential oil

Procedure:

1. Melt the beeswax or Shea or cocoa butter in a saucepan.

2. Remove from the heat and add the oil. Mix well.

3. Mix in the essential oil then pour into your container. Allow to cool before using.

Essential Oil Wrinkle Reducing Facial Oil

Ingredients:

- ¼ cup coconut, almond or jojoba oil (normal skin), or olive, argan or avocado oil (dry skin) or grape seed oil (oily skin)
- 5 drops of lavender, patchouli, sandalwood, chamomile or rose essential oil

Procedure:

1. Pour the oil into a glass bottle.

2. Add the essential oil and shake to mix well.

Facial Scrub

(Use this if you prefer physical exfoliation, i.e. using grainy substances, rather than acids to exfoliate your face.)

Ingredients:

- 1 tablespoon coconut, almond or jojoba oil (normal skin), or olive, argan or avocado oil (dry skin) or grape seed oil (oily skin)
- 1 teaspoon fine sugar, oatmeal or cornmeal (you need to experiment on what works best for your skin, but avoid salt for facial skin even if it is finely ground since it is too harsh.)

Procedure:

1. Mix everything together in a small bowl.

2. Apply this on your clean face with your fingertips. Use circular motions. Do not scrub one area of the face for longer than 2 seconds.

3. Exfoliate your face for 1 minute or longer but not more than 2 minutes.

4. If your skin becomes red or inflamed, you either pressed too hard, exfoliated too long or need to change your choice of grainy scrub.

Facial Exfoliating Mask

(This uses chemical exfoliation through the acids in the ingredients to dissolve the dead skin cells.)

Ingredients:

- 4 tablespoons of yoghurt
- 1 tablespoon fresh lemon juice
- 1 tablespoon crushed fresh strawberries

Procedure:

1. Combine everything in a bowl.

2. Apply to your clean face but avoid the eye area.

3. Leave on for 15-20 minutes, then wash off.

Yoghurt and Sugar Exfoliating Scrub and Mask

(This combines physical and chemical exfoliation.)

Ingredients:

- 4 tablespoons yoghurt
- 1 tablespoon fine sugar
  Optional: 1 teaspoon honey

Procedure:

1. Combine everything in a bowl and apply to your face.

2. Use your fingertips to scrub the sugar all over but avoid the eye area.

3. After a minute of scrubbing, leave the mask on for 15-20 minutes, then rinse it off.

Vitamin C Moisturizer

(Since vitamin C is an antioxidant, this can replace the antioxidant moisturizer described above. Keep this in an opaque container since light can oxidize vitamin C and render it useless.)

Ingredients:

- 1 teaspoon of crushed vitamin C tablets
- 2 ounces of distilled water in an opaque bottle
- ¼ cup coconut, almond or jojoba oil (normal skin), or olive, argan or avocado oil (dry skin) or grape seed oil (oily skin)
- ¼ cup beeswax (normal or oily skin) or shea or cocoa butter (dry skin)

Procedure:

1. Dissolve the crushed vitamin C in the water. Set aside.

2. Melt the beeswax or Shea or cocoa butter in a saucepan.

3. Remove from the heat then add the oil. Mix well.

4. When the mixture has slightly cooled, add the vitamin C water and quickly mix everything together.

5. Pour into your container.

6. Cover the container immediately even if the mixture is still warm. When using this, get a pea-sized amount then quickly cover the jar to avoid product oxidation. Keep this in the refrigerator.

Conclusion

Thank you again for purchasing this book!

I hope this book was able to help you to know how to prevent and minimize wrinkles with natural, homemade skin care products.

The next step is to try out the recipes listed here and see what works for you.

Finally, if you enjoyed this book, please take the time to share your thoughts and post a positive review on Amazon. It'd be greatly appreciated!

In addition, please remember to LIKE our Facebook page in order to find other resources and upcoming promotions:

https://www.facebook.com/joypublishing

With sincere thanks,

SOFIE KING

FAST HAIR GROWTH FOR BEGINNERS

Natural Hair Growth Secrets and Hair Loss Cure for Growing Long and Fast Hair

SOFIE KING

Table of Contents

Introduction

I want to thank you and congratulate you for purchasing the book, "**Fast Hair Growth for Beginners**: *Natural Hair Growth Secrets and Hair Loss Cure for Growing Long and Fast Hair*".

This book contains proven steps and strategies on how to grow beautiful and strong hair fast and help cure hair loss using natural methods.

In this book, you will be taught the correct ways to cleanse, condition and care for your hair in order to minimize breakage and promote fast hair growth. You will also learn about the right nutrition to help promote strong hair. Some hair loss cures will also be provided to you. Lastly, you will find some easy do it yourself hair mask recipes that you can try at home.

Thanks again for purchasing this book, I hope you enjoy it! Please take some time to stop by and LIKE our Facebook page:

https://www.facebook.com/joypublishing

With gratitude,

SOFIE KING

Chapter 1

Hair Growth Facts

What do you think of the state of your hair right now? Is it thick or thin? Is it treated or natural? Does it feel soft and smooth or brittle and dull? The current state of your hair will determine how fast and how long the strands can grow.

The truth is that human hair generally grows at the same rate, which is approximately half of a millimetre every day, which means that your hair becomes half an inch longer every month. The healthier and younger you are, the faster your hair can grow out. Apart from that, your genetics and hormones are additional natural factors that play a major role in hair growth. Other factors would be the hair treatments that you choose, the everyday hair care products that you use, your nutritional intake and even the condition of your scalp.

Since your goal is to have long and beautiful hair, you should aim to protect it from anything that will impede it from growing out at its normal rate. Likewise, you should "feed" it the right nutrients and make an extra effort to protect and take care of it to ensure that it will not be damaged as it continues to grow. After all, the only thing that is stopping your hair from growing fast is if it is harmed in some way.

How Hair Grows?

In order to understand the nature of hair growth, let us take a look at the three phases that describe this natural process: the anagen phase, the catagen phase, and the telogen phase.

The anagen phase is the moment when hair pushes itself out from the follicle. It is the time when the hair is in the middle of the growth process. When the hair slowly detaches itself from the follicle and "dies", this is the catagen phase. Finally, it would reach the telogen phase when it is pushed out from the follicle and is shed off by the body.

Of course, not all of the hair on the scalp go through the phases at the same time. As new strands of hair are produced each day, old strands are shed off. New hair replaces old hair every day, which makes it a cycle.

However, the moment when old hair is *not* replaced by new hair, then hair loss takes place. This is a problem that many people, both men and women, face. Since it is such a common issue, many companies have tried to come up with a cure-all that promises to promote hair growth and hair loss. But keep in mind that hair will not grow out fast and long within a few weeks. No such product can do that, and anything that claims that it can actually means they can help keep the hair stay strong as it continues to grow out naturally.

Fortunately, there are plenty of ways on how you can get the hair that you have always wanted. As we all know, each person's physiological makeup is different, which is why not all remedies and tips work for everyone. The bottom-line is that you should do your best to keep your hair and scalp healthy, and in return you will get the best hair that your body can produce.

Chapter 2

The Correct Ways to Cleanse and Condition Hair

When someone says "fast" in hair growth, what it actually means is that you provide the right conditions for your hair to grow out without risk of breakage. It also means that you nourish your body with the right nutrients so that it will continue to let your hair grow out without disruption because it does not lack the necessary vitamins and minerals in doing so.

In order to promote fast hair growth, you would need to develop some healthy habits and make a few changes in your choice of hair care products and styling techniques:

Use a Shampoo and Conditioner that Do Not Contain Harmful Chemicals

The funny thing about many drugstore shampoos is, although they promise to help care for your hair, they actually contain harmful chemicals that will ultimately damage your hair. These shampoos and conditioners contain ingredients that are meant to prolong their shelf life or kill dandruff-causing bacteria. Unfortunately, both thin down the hair because they are too strong for your scalp and cause skin irritation; and when your scalp is unhealthy, it is only natural for the hair that grows out of it to be unhealthy, too.

There are two chemical surfactants that you need to avoid in shampoos and conditioners, and these are sodium lauryl sulfate or SLS and sodium laureth sulfate or SLES. They are responsible for producing lather or foam to make the shampoo seem more economical because even just a small amount can easily be spread across the hair. However, these are highly toxic and reported by the Environmental Working Group to cause skin irritation, organ toxicity and cancer.

Two other harmful ingredients in many shampoos are isopropyl alcohol and propylene glycol. They are added to shampoos that help combat oily hair due to their "drying" effects that make you feel clean afterward. However, it is so strong that it will strip away the natural oils and proteins that keep the hair from becoming brittle. Continuous use will cause the hair to become thin or to break sooner than normal.

There is yet another compound that you need to look out for in shampoos, and it is labelled as diethanomaline or DEA. Sometimes it is listed as Cocamide DEA or Lauramide DEA under the list of ingredients. It is added to hair products because it makes the product feel creamy. However, constantly using this product can cause cancer, especially if you use it with other cosmetic products. The DEA reacts with the nitrites found in these products and turn into nitrosamines, which is a carcinogenic compound, according to the International Agency for Research on Cancer.

Do plenty of research online for shampoos and conditioners that are guaranteed to be free from these harmful chemicals. Read reviews on these brands and then purchase sample sizes to try for yourself. In most cases, a mild shampoo and conditioner are all you need to gently wash off dirt and excess oil from your hair yet maintain the natural oils that keep your hair smooth and strong.

Always Condition your Hair after Shampooing

The basic role of shampoo is to strip away the dirt and oil that have accumulated in your hair. This will help prevent your scalp from becoming irritated and developing dandruff, and it also makes your hair feel smooth and clean instead of greasy.

However, since shampoos are designed to get rid of oil, it is only normal for it to remove the natural oils that are keeping our hair healthy as well. This is where the conditioner comes in.

A conditioner is basically an emollient that will restore the protective oils in your hair. The next time you shampoo your hair, notice how it feels rough and dry afterwards. Then, after you condition your hair notice how silky the texture is as a consequence. Skipping the conditioner will put your hair at risk of breakage because it will still take time for your scalp to produce the oils that will moisturize your hair again.

It is best to choose the conditioner that pairs with your shampoo. Manufacturers have special formulas that complement a brand of shampoo and conditioner together. You would want to maximize their features to help keep your hair strong for faster hair growth.

Learn How to Wash your Hair the Right Way

There is actually a correct technique on how to wash your hair. By learning this technique, you can prevent hair loss due to breakage and even dandruff. That is because the correct way to wash your hair involves keeping your scalp clean as well. Just make sure to use the right type of shampoo and conditioner in order to ensure clean and moisturized hair.

The first step in washing your hair and scalp is to wet it thoroughly. Make sure that it is fully soaked with water by pointing the shower nozzle directly on your head.

Next is to apply shampoo onto your hair and scalp. Here is an economical way of spreading shampoo across your hair and scalp without using too much product: fill a small bottle (approximately 2 and a half inches in length and 1 and a half inches in diameter) three-quarters of the way with water and then squeeze out a desired amount of shampoo into the bottle. After that, shake the bottle vigorously and squeeze out the mixture across your scalp. Never apply or squeeze out shampoo onto a single section of your scalp each time, especially if you are using strong shampoo because it might thin down the hair in that section.

Once you have applied shampoo, massage your scalp with the pads of your fingers. Be careful not to let your nails dig into your scalp for this might harm the delicate skin and put it at risk for infection. Massage in gentle circular motions, starting with the top of the head and moving your way out to the back of your ears and your nape. The goal is to disturb the deep-seated dirt and oil on the scalp so that these will get washed away during the rinse. Let the shampoo sit in your hair for approximately a minute or two before rinsing away.

If your hair gets tangled easily, you can apply a bit of conditioner before shampooing. Put a small amount of product on the palm of your hand and then rub your hands together. Gently apply the conditioner onto the tangled sections of hair and leave it on for a minute or two; you can proceed with washing your face while waiting. Then, rinse off the conditioner thoroughly and move on to shampoo.

After you have shampooed and rinsed your hair thoroughly, you can now proceed to restore the moisture in your hair by applying conditioner. You will only need to condition the tips of your hair, or the lower half of your strands, not the entire head of hair. That's because after you step out of the bathroom, your scalp will gradually produce the natural oils in your hair within hours, which will be distributed across your roots, but not necessarily all the way to the tips especially if you have short hair. This makes conditioning your hair from root to tip a bad idea because it will only leave you with incredibly greasy roots.

To apply conditioner, squeeze a small amount on the palm of your hand and then rub your palms together. Then, rub the product onto the tips of your hair. You can do this by rubbing the hair tips in between your palms to distribute the product evenly. After that, let the product sit in your hair for three to five minutes, or as based on the manufacturer's instructions. You can wash the rest of your body while waiting. If you have long hair, wrap your hair into a shower cap so that the conditioner will not spread across your neck and back.

Rinse your hair thoroughly after that. The best way to rinse your hair would be to bend your head down before wetting it. This will prevent the product from trickling down your neck and back as you rinse. A major cause of acne is the use of hair products, after all.

Make sure to rinse your hair well enough until the water runs clear. Then, wrap your head with a hair towel to dry. Be careful not to wrap it too tightly. If you are not comfortable wearing a hair towel, place a towel across your shoulders to catch the water dripping from your newly washed hair.

Deep Condition your Hair Once a Week

To keep your hair strong as you continue to let it grow out, it is a good idea to deep condition it or use a hair mask. A deep conditioner will help strengthen your hair and preventing breakage. Keep in mind that deep conditioners cannot reverse damage. Hair is made up of dead cells, which means that they are unable to regenerate and restore themselves back to their previous state, unlike skin. What a deep conditioner will do is to keep the hair from becoming further damaged.

There are plenty of deep conditioning products on the market. Once again, choose the ones that do not contain any of the harmful chemicals mentioned earlier. You can also whip up your own hair masks using natural ingredients. See chapter 6 for some recipes that you can try.

Chapter 3

Change your Hair Habits

Little habits have major effects in the long run, and hair care is not exempted from this principle. The length, condition and volume of your hair will depend a lot on how you treat it on a regular basis.

To help you with fast hair growth, here is a list of everyday hair care habits that you need to start making or breaking:

Never Comb your Hair while It Is Wet

Hair and scalp are at its weakest state when it is wet, therefore combing will easily cause the hair root to dislodge from the follicle. After bathing, let your hair dry in room temperature. You can also blow dry it under cool or low warm setting if you are in a hurry, but make sure to do this sparingly.

Avoid Dying your Hair

Plenty of hair dyes on the market contain harmful chemicals that can harm not just your hair and scalp, but your entire body as well. Here is a list of these chemicals:

- *PPD or P-phenylenediamine*. This causes bladder cancer and is toxic to the immune and nervous system including the lungs and the kidney. It also causes long term asthma.

- **_Persulfates_**. This is an ingredient in strong bleach and will irritate your scalp. It also causes asthma and lung damage.

- **_Resorcinol_**. This is a chemical that disrupts the endocrine system. It causes hypothyroidism, depression, and nausea.

- **_Hydrogen Peroxide_**. This chemical has corrosive properties meant to bleach hair, but it also causes hair brittleness. It is extremely toxic and can cause cancer if used repeatedly.

- **_Ammonia_**. This chemical will irritate your scalp and trigger an asthma attack. However, it is often used as an alternative to PPD in many hair dye products because it is less harmful.

- **_Lead Acetate_**. This is a harmful chemical that is meant to darken hair. However, it is extremely toxic to both the brain and the nervous system so avoid it at all costs.

- **_4-ABP_**. This extremely carcinogenic chemical is often a by-product of the hair dye process, particularly if you want to dye your hair black, blonde or red.

Avoid dyeing your hair with products that contain any of these chemicals. Even a single use of hair dye products can cause brittleness and thinness, which eventually leads to breakage. If possible, resort to more natural methods of changing your hair color. You can try two of the recipes mentioned in Chapter 6 for darkening or lightening your hair.

Do Not Use Elastics and Other Tight Hair Clips and Bands

Continuous use of hair bands, hair clips and bobby pins will pull your hair at the roots, weakening them and speeding up shedding.

If you have long hair and you do not like the feeling of it sticking to your neck during hot weather or falling across your shoulders and back, then use a hair clamp instead. This will hold your hair up without pulling it at the roots because all you have to do is to put your hair up into a loose twist and clamp it.

If you cannot help using hair bands and hair clips, then what you can do is to avoid tying your hair up from the same angle. Doing so will repeatedly pull certain hairs from their roots and eventually cause shedding. Try to add variety in where you place your pony tail, such as going for a side ponytail or pigtails. You can also put your hair into a loose braid every now and then to prevent the band from pulling tightly at your hair.

Shield your Scalp from Direct Sunlight

Many people tend to forego applying sunscreen on their scalp, but doing so will put the scalp at risk for developing sunburn and infection. This will have an effect on the hair follicles on the scalp as well, causing them to weaken and shed hair fast. Prolonged sunlight exposure can also damage the hair and cause brittleness, then breakage.

Use a hat to cover your hair if you are to become exposed to sunlight for extended lengths of time. You can also use a dark-colored umbrella to further shield your skin and scalp from the sun. It is also a good idea to regularly use scalp and hair sunblock, which usually come in the form of sprays and lotions.

Minimize your Use of Hot Tools

Flat and curling irons and even blow dryers will damage your hair, especially if you use them on a regular basis. The heat causes the hair to become dry and brittle, making the strands easily prone to breakage and split ends. Limit your use of hot tools to twice a month and always use a heat protectant spray or serum whenever you do to minimize the effects of the heat.

Chapter 4

Proper Nutrition for Healthy Hair Growth

What you feed your body will definitely affect the health of your hair. It will take a few months for a poor diet to cause weak and thin hair, but it will also take months of following a healthy diet before new hair grows out it its best state. This means you should start making changes in your diet as soon as possible so that you can support fast hair growth for months to come.

Proper nutrition for the sake of healthy hair growth involves eating nutrients that make hair follicles strong as they come out of the scalp. It is important to stop unhealthy habits that will counteract the effects of these nutrients as well, such as smoking and inadequate sleep.

Here are the top 10 nutrients that you need to eat regularly in order to have strong hair that will grow out fast:

- *Protein*

    One of the most important nutrients for fast hair growth is protein. In fact, hair itself is made of dead protein. This nutrient can be obtained from eggs, fish, wheat germ, poultry, milk, tofu, nuts, legumes and yogurt.

    Protein is made up of building blocks called amino acids. After consuming protein, the digestive system breaks it down into amino acids, which is them absorbed into the bloodstream and distributed throughout the cells of the body to help create antibodies, hormones, enzymes, blood cells and body tissue, including hair follicles.

- ***Vitamin D***

  Vitamin D is a fat-soluble vitamin that you can get from fatty fish and fortified foods, but your body can only make use of when the skin gets a healthy amount of exposure to sunlight.

  Lack of vitamin D in the body is one of the most common factors for hair loss. A study that was published in the 2011 issue of Clinical, Cosmetic Investigative Dermatology showed that low levels of vitamin D is responsible for female-pattern hair loss as well as the condition called Telogen effluvium, which is hair loss due to excessive shedding.

- ***Omega-3 Fatty Acids***

  Omega-3 fatty acids are vital to human healthy, partly because it reduces inflammation and hair loss. There are three essential types of omega-3 that you will need for the growth of your hair, and these are DHA or docosahexaenoic acid, EPA or eicosapentaenoic acid, and ALA or alpha-linolenic acid. You can get them from vegetable oils such as olive oil and sesame oil, nuts and seeds (such as walnuts and flaxseeds) as well as oily fish (such as salmon and tuna) and fish oil supplements.

  Not getting enough omega-3 fatty acids in your diet is partially responsible for hair loss, according to a study conducted by the University of Maryland Medical Center. In order to boost fast hair growth and minimize hair loss and breakage, it is important to take one to two capsules of fish oil every day. This will prevent dandruff or flaky scalp and minimize inflammation as well.

- ***Biotin***

  Biotin is so potent for strengthening hair that you will find plenty of biotin supplements on the market specifically for hair growth. Biotin is a B vitamin that helps promote body growth, including healthy hair. Deficiency in the vitamin will lead to brittle hair and unhealthy skin.

  Biotin is often prescribed to help treat alopecia or hair loss in both children and adults, and it is known to be most effective if paired with zinc. The great thing about biotin is that it will not only promote hair growth, but also improve hair volume. You can obtain biotin from foods such as chicken eggs, carrots, Swiss chard, onions, cucumbers, cauliflower, strawberries and raspberries, goat's milk, cow's milk, almonds and walnuts, and halibut. You can also take it in supplement form, with a maximum of 30 mg per day.

- ***Vitamin E***

  More and more experts are calling vitamin E as a beauty vitamin because it helps improve the condition of the skin and hair. Although more studies need to be conducted in order to explain the effects of vitamin E on hair, experts agree that it promotes healthy hair growth and helps prevent hair loss by boosting the growth of capillaries in the scalp. The good news about vitamin E is that it also has the potential to slow down aging, which includes premature greying.

  To maximize the effects of vitamin E, it is advised that you take it internally as part of your diet and externally by applying vitamin E oil onto your scalp. Some of the best sources of vitamin E are green leafy vegetables (such as spinach, collards, kale, Swiss chards and mustard greens), seeds such as almonds, avocado, papaya, and kiwi. You can also take it in supplement form, but make sure to limit it to 15 to 19 mg (or 22.5 to 28.5 I.U.) for each day.

● *Iron*

Iron deficiency is one of the leading causes of hair loss. Likewise, proper intake of iron will help treat and prevent hair loss. Iron is a mineral that is naturally found in the body, particularly in hemoglobin. This can be found in red blood cells and is responsible for transporting oxygen throughout the cells in the body.

There are two types of dietary iron, and they are heme iron and non-heme iron. Heme iron can be obtained from animal products such as poultry, fish and beef. It is the type that the body can easily absorb. Non-heme iron can be found in plant products such as whole grain, beans, lentils, spinach and fortified cereals. It is not as easy to absorb.

You can take iron in the form of supplements with no more than 8 mg for men and 10 mg for women over 18 years old. It is best to take iron with vitamin C to boost absorption. Avoid drinking tea and milk while taking iron for the tannins in tea and the calcium in milk will prevent full absorption of non-heme iron.

● *Selenium and Zinc*

Hair loss happens when hair becomes thinner, dry and brittle. To help prevent these three symptoms, it is essential to have regularly include the minerals selenium and zinc in your diet. These two help promote healthy hair growth and prevent hair loss.

Deficiency in selenium slows down the ability of the hair follicle to produce hair while deficiency in zinc weakens the immune system and increases the risk for infections that can contribute to hair loss. Selenium is an antioxidant that helps the body cleanse, while zinc strengthens the hair follicles.

You can obtain selenium from foods such as garlic, liver, whole grains, butter and fish. It can also be taken in supplement form with a dosage of 25 to 50 mcg per day.

Zinc can be obtained from red meat, poultry, oysters, shellfish, whole grains and legumes. It can be taken as a supplement as well, with no more than 15 mcg per day. It is best to take zinc along with protein foods to maximize absorption.

- ### *Vitamin B5 or Pantothenic Acid*

Pantothenic acid is very common in hair products because it helps strengthen hair follicles and prevent hair loss. The main function of this essential vitamin is that it helps the body in metabolizing protein and fats. This will help your hair follicles to absorb the amino acids in protein more efficiently, leading to the growth of strong hair. Furthermore, this vitamin helps prevent the symptoms of dandruff, which are flaking and skin itching. As you know, a healthy scalp is important in promoting fast hair growth.

You will be able to get pantothenic acid from whole grains, vegetables, legumes, fish and meats. You can also take it in supplement form along with other B complex vitamins. The recommended daily dosage of this vitamin is a maximum of 5 mg for those over 19 years old. However, keep in mind that the vitamin B5 supplement is not recommended for people with hemophilia for it may counteract with certain medications.

Chapter 5

Hair Loss Cures

Up until now, science is yet to find a cure for complete hair loss. The best thing that a person who is suffering from hair loss and balding can do is to find ways to strengthen the hair that they have left, stimulate new hair growth, and to minimize further hair loss.

It is a natural part of the aging process to have thinning hair. Excessive hair loss, however, is caused by genetic and environmental factors including diet and use of products that contain harmful chemicals.

If you apply all of the natural methods that have been discussed in the previous chapters, you are already minimizing hair loss and promoting new hair growth. However, if natural methods do not work, then you will have to resort to the use of prescription and over-the-counter drugs.

Minoxidil is a common medication for androgenetic alopecia, which is also called pattern baldness, and alopecia areata, or hair loss due to autoimmune issues. It is available as over the counter and prescription, although the latter is obviously more potent. This treatment comes in the form of liquid or foam and is applied directly onto the scalp. Hair growth from minoxidil will be thinner and not grow as long as normal hair, but it is enough to cover bald spots. It will take at least three months before effects are noticeable.

Steroid hormones, such as corticosteroids, is another form of treatment for hair loss, particularly alopecia areata. It is injected into the scalp each month or taken in pill form. Corticosteroids in the form of topical ointments are also available, but are not as effective.

For hair loss caused by skin problems such as psoriasis, Anthralin is often used as treatment. This prescription medication is available in ointment form and is applied directly to the scalp to stimulate the hair follicles to produce hair. It will take at least 3 months before any effects can be seen.

For male pattern baldness, the oral prescription medication Finasteride is used. It helps promote new hair growth by extending the anagen phase.

If all else fails, you can turn to surgical methods such as hair transplants. Hair, along with its roots, are surgically removed from other parts of the body or part of the scalp and then transplanted to the more prominent bald spots on top of the head. It may take several sessions before the treatment is completed. Also, it does not prove to be effective for everyone.

Keep in mind that these treatments should only be a "last resort." In most cases, changes in diet and hair care habits are enough to help slow down hair loss and promote the growth of stronger hair.

Chapter 6

Do it Yourself Hair Care Recipes

Here are some very effective and easy to make hair care recipes that you can create at home for your weekly deep conditioning and scalp treatments:

Scalp Exfoliating Scrub
For the prevention of dandruff caused by product build-up

Ingredients:

- 1 Tbsp. brown sugar
- 3 Tbsp. coconut butter (or your favorite conditioner)

Procedure:

1. Wash and clean hair with shampoo. Rinse thoroughly.

2. Combine both ingredients into a small bowl until you get a thick paste.

3. Apply scrub gently onto the scalp and massage in a light circular motion. Start with the nape and move upward.

4. Rinse hair thoroughly and condition as usual.

Herbal Rinse

Best applied after using heavy hair styling products to get rid of product build-up

Ingredients:

- 4 Tbsp. vinegar (preferably apple cider vinegar)
- 1 herbal tea bag (sage, chamomile, mint or nettle)
- 1 to 2 drops of therapeutic-grade essential oil (lavender, peppermint, rosemary, cedar wood or clary sage)

Procedure:

1. Heat vinegar in a glass or ceramic pan over low heat until steaming, but not boiling.

2. Steep tea bag in hot vinegar for a minimum of 15 minutes.

3. Add essential oil to the mixture.

4. Wash and clean hair with shampoo. Rinse thoroughly.

5. Carefully apply the herbal rinse onto the hair in gentle rubbing motions. Wrap in shower cap and let sit for 5 to 8 minutes. Rinse thoroughly.

Butter Deep Conditioner
To help minimize split ends

Ingredients:

- 1 Tbsp. Shea butter
- 1 Tbsp. coconut butter (or your favorite conditioner)
- 1/2 Tbsp. olive oil (or jojoba or meadow foam oil)

Procedure:

1. Soften Shea butter by leaving it in room temperature or under direct sunlight for 5 to 10 minutes or until soft.

2. Combine the Shea butter with the coconut butter and oil. Set aside to cool until hard. Stir well if the oils start to separate.

3. Wet hair thoroughly and apply the paste to the ends. Let sit for 15 to 20 minutes. Rinse thoroughly afterward. If hair is long, pin it up with a hair clamp to prevent the butter from touching your neck and back.

Name of Recipe Avocado Deep Conditioner
For all hair types

Ingredients:

- 1 to 2 Tbsp. avocado meat (depending on length of hair)
- 1 Tbsp. coconut butter (or your favorite conditioner)

Procedure:

1. Mash the avocado and mix together with coconut butter in a bowl.

2. Apply the mixture to the hair from root to tip. Wrap hair with shower cap. It is even better if you wrap it in a damp towel that was soaked in hot water before wrapping with a shower cap.

3. Let sit for 20 minutes before rinsing off thoroughly.

4. Blow dry hair using low setting to open up the hair shafts and promote further absorption of avocado oils.

Coffee Conditioner
Best for conditioning dark hair

Ingredients:

- 2 Tbsp. pure coffee granules
- 1 Tbsp. boiling water
- 2 Tbsp. coconut butter (or your favorite conditioner)

Procedure:

1. Wash and clean hair with shampoo. Rinse thoroughly.

2. In a bowl, mix the coffee granules and coconut butter.

3. Add boiling water and mix to create a paste.

4. Apply onto the tips of the hair and cover with shower cap. Let sit for 20 minutes before rinsing.

Hair Brightening Conditioner
For light brown or blonde hair

Ingredients:

- 6 tea bags of organic chamomile
- 1/2 cup plain yogurt
- 1 to 2 Tbsp. pure honey
- 7 drops of therapeutic-grade lavender essential oil
- 1 cup water

Procedure:

1. Boil water and then steep tea bags in it for 15 minutes. Throw away teabags afterward.

2. Mix the yogurt, honey, and lavender oil together with the chamomile tea.

3. Carefully apply the mixture onto dry hair, from root to tips.

4. Wrap hair in shower cap and let sit for at least 30 minutes.

5. Rinse off thoroughly and shampoo hair.

Conclusion

Thank you again for purchasing this book!

I hope this book was able to help you to grow strong and beautiful hair fast.

The next step is to continue to take good care of your hair and scalp. Minimize the use of harmful products and techniques that will cause breakage. Also, eat nutritious foods that will enable your body to produce strong and thick hair.

Finally, if you enjoyed this book, please take the time to share your thoughts and post a positive review on Amazon. It'd be greatly appreciated!

In addition, please remember to check out our Facebook page in order to find other resources and upcoming promotions:

https://www.facebook.com/joypublishing

With sincere thanks,

SOFIE KING

One Last Thing...

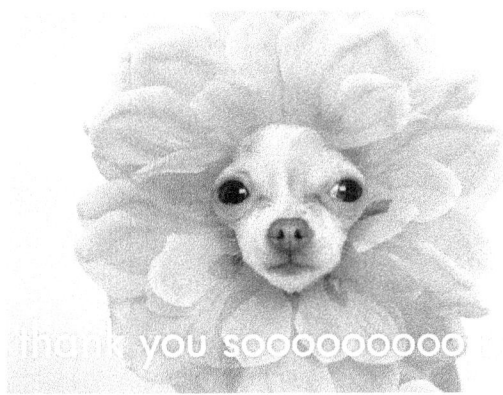

If you believe that this book is worth sharing, would you please take the time to let others know how it affected your life? If it turns out to make a difference in the lives of others, they will be forever grateful to you, as will I.